Firas Maalej
Amal Samet
Meriam Triki

Thyroid nodules

Firas Maalej
Amal Samet
Meriam Triki

Thyroid nodules

Cytohistological correlation

ScienciaScripts

Imprint
Any brand names and product names mentioned in this book are subject to trademark, brand or patent protection and are trademarks or registered trademarks of their respective holders. The use of brand names, product names, common names, trade names, product descriptions etc. even without a particular marking in this work is in no way to be construed to mean that such names may be regarded as unrestricted in respect of trademark and brand protection legislation and could thus be used by anyone.

Cover image: www.ingimage.com

This book is a translation from the original published under ISBN 978-620-6-72044-7.

Publisher:
Sciencia Scripts
is a trademark of
Dodo Books Indian Ocean Ltd. and OmniScriptum S.R.L publishing group

120 High Road, East Finchley, London, N2 9ED, United Kingdom
Str. Armeneasca 28/1, office 1, Chisinau MD-2012, Republic of Moldova, Europe
Printed at: see last page
ISBN: 978-620-8-04211-0

PLAN

INTRODUCTION

A thyroid nodule is a localised enlargement of the thyroid tissue. It is clinically palpable in 5 to 7% of the adult population and histologically present in 50% according to autopsy data [1]. These nodules are usually benign, but clinically palpable nodules may represent thyroid cancer in around 4% to 6.5% of cases [2]. The distinction between benign and malignant nodules has always posed the main problem for clinicians. To this day, there are no clinical, biological or radiological arguments that allow a formal distinction to be made between benign and malignant nodules. Management of thyroid nodules therefore essentially involves assessing the potential for malignancy, and must be multidisciplinary, involving endocrinologists, pathologists, radiologists, isotopists and ENT surgeons.In this context, diagnostic strategies have gradually been developed, based on the analysis of a number of factors: data from the interview and clinical examination and the results of paraclinical investigations, in order to operate only on suspected nodules. Within these different diagnostic strategies, fine needle aspiration (FNA) now occupies a place of its own alongside scintigraphy and ultrasound.CPAF is a rapid, simple, inexpensive, non-invasive and reliable technique for identifying thyroid nodules that are malignant or suspected of being malignant, avoiding unnecessary systematic surgery in a high percentage of cases, and providing a high level of safety. select patients for surgery. Recent studies have shown the superiority of CPAF over other diagnostic methods and have highlighted its ability to differentiate frequent but benign colloid or macrovascular lesions from lesions suspected of malignancy, the exact nature of which can only be confirmed by histological study [2]. In 1995, thanks to the development of the method and the experience of cytopathologists and sampling physicians, the Agence Nationale pour le Développement et de l'Evaluation Médicale (ANDEM) confirmed the role of thyroid cytopuncture in the management of thyroid nodules [3].

1 FINE NEEDLE ASPIRATION (FNA)

1.1 History

The technique of CPAF of a thyroid nodule is a very old one, described as far back as 1930 by Martin and Ellis [4], at the time using large needles. Subsequently, Silverman [5] introduced the Tru-Cut technique using tissue biopsy needles. None of these techniques has been widely used because of the fear of dissemination of the malignant process during puncture, the high number of false negatives and the often serious complications. In the 1950s, Scandinavian investigators, in particular Esselstyn and Cryle [6], became familiar with fine needle aspiration and this technique became the reference diagnostic method for Anglo-Saxon authors. Since 1995, this technique has become increasingly used under the impetus of authors such as Bonneau and Zajdela in 1964, who helped to establish its superiority over other diagnostic methods in the investigation of thyroid nodules [7, 8]. In 1995, the ANDEM confirmed the role of thyroid cytopuncture in the management of thyroid nodules when it published its recommendations [3].

Thanks to the development of the method and the experience of the cytologists and samplers, CPAF is now definitively putting aside thyroid puncture-biopsy performed with large-bore trocars. CPAF is recognised as a reliable, inexpensive, non-invasive method of studying thyroid nodules that is superior in quality to puncture-biopsy, thus allowing better selection of patients for surgery [9].

1.2 Technical

1.2.1Patient position

The patient lies supine, with the neck hyperextended and a block under the shoulders; this position ensures better exposure of the thyroid and accessibility to both poles. Local anaesthetic is usually unnecessary, as the puncture is virtually painless.

1.2.2Echo-guided technique

Ultrasound guidance is performed using a linear diagnostic ultrasound probe or a micro-convex vascular probe (6 to 8 mhz). The technique currently used is freehand puncture without a guide, with the operator checking that the needle (which is not attached to the probe) has been correctly inserted into the thyroid parenchyma. The probe must be sterile after disinfection of the neck, and the contact agent should preferably be sterile water, as any trace of gel that might be carried back by the needle with the sample could render it illegible after staining.At present, most teams use the CPAF with a needle gauge of ranging from 23 to 27 Gauges [10].

1.2.3 sampling technique

The current reference technique is the non-aspirated capillary technique, first described in France by Zajdela in 1987 [11], and recommended in the most recent guidelines [12].The needle is placed in the thyroid nodule under ultrasound guidance, so that the bevel of the needle can be seen at all times. The sampler applies small axial rotation and back-and-forth movements in several axes for a few seconds, while continuously checking that the "tip-echo" remains in the nodule: this is known as radial cytopuncture. These movements are maintained until a serosa rises in the tip of the needle; one or two slides are obtained at each passage and 2 to 3 punctures are performed at the level of each nodule.

Larger-bore needles can be used for the slow evacuation of predominantly liquid nodules, by aspirating with a syringe fitted to the needle. At the end of the cytopuncture, the sampling site must be compressed. performed to prevent the formation of any haematomas.

1.2.4Spreading

The product of the thyroid puncture is deposited and spread on 2 or 3 dry slides, then the sampler spreads it out, which must be done very carefully to avoid crushing the cells while respecting their arrangement. There must be at least 6 slides; the patient's name and the nodule identification number must be written on the frosted side of the slide to avoid any possible errors. The choice of cytological technique is the responsibility of the cytopathologist; the most commonly used stain is haematoxylin and eosin, which provides a good balance between slide legibility, cost, speed of execution and an overall view of morphology and cell structure [13]. In the case of fluid samples, the paraffin embedding of the cell pellet allows additional immunohistochemical techniques to be carried out according to the methods developed on the paraffin-embedded tissue; immunohistochemical techniques can also be carried out on samples from cell spreads stored at -20°C or from monolayer spreads. Finally, certain data (clinical, biological, ultrasound) must be specified on the request form that accompanies the thyroid cytopuncture product to the laboratory to ensure a reliable cytopathological interpretation [14] (Table I).

Table I: Information to be provided on the cytopunction

Essential clinical, biological or ultrasound information, or useful for reliable cytological interpretation	
Essential information Location of nodule(s) Size of nodule(s) Context of hypothyroidism, autoimmune thyroiditis or basedow's disease Presence of antithyroid antibodies Previous treatment with radioactive iodine Previous cervical irradiation Personal history of cancer	Useful information Results of any previous cytopuncture Concomitant treatment with thyroid hormones TSH levels Results of thyroid ultrasound scan

1.2.5 Precautions

CPAF is a harmless procedure for which there are few contraindications, essentially major haemostasis disorders. It can be performed in patients taking acetosalicylic acid (ASA) without increasing the risk of bleeding. The risk of bleeding is reduced up to a daily dose of 100 mg of ASA, and patients receiving higher doses should stop treatment for 10 days before the procedure [15]. In patients taking VKAs (Coumadin, Phenprocoumone), it is recommended that doses be adjusted until INR =< 1.5 with a relay with heparin. For patients taking antiplatelet agents (Clopidogrel, Ticlopidine), the treatment must be taken more than 24 hours before the operation. For oral anticoagulants, treatment must be stopped 48 hours before the operation for Dabigatran (72 hours if renal function is impaired and up to 94 hours without bypass if end-stage renal failure, 24 hours for Rivaroxaban and 24 to 48 hours for Apixaban.

1.3 Criteria for validity

The number of samples: 3 different punctures are generally recommended for each nodule [16]. The number of cell sheets per slide: the authors consider that there must be at least 06 cell sheets (each containing at least 10 well visualised follicular cells: well stained, well fixed and undistorted) on at least 02 slides from different punctures for a sample to be considered benign [17]. In this context, punctures that do not provide sufficient material are said to be uninterpretable or blank, and this is an indication for repeat cytopuncture. In half of all cases, sufficient material is obtained from the second sample, but in some cases, despite taking several samples, insufficient material may be obtained, especially if a cystic or sclerotic lesion is present. The puncture must not be haemorrhagic: the total absence of red blood cells is very difficult in practice; there is no recognised figure in the literature. of red blood cells above which the slide is considered uninterpretable, but it is It is recognised that a haemorrhagic puncture must be repeated at a distance.

1.4 Indications

Several recommendations have been published in recent years in Europe and the United States specifying the indications for CPAF in the case of a thyroid nodule [18, 19, 20]. These recommendations are based on stratification of the risk of clinical and ultrasound malignancy. In this context, in 2017 the European Thyroid Association (ETA) proposed an algorithm specifying the indications for CPAF according to ultrasound data, the EU-TIRADS classification and the size of the nodule (Figure 1); thus cytopuncture is indicated for [21]:

- Nodules > 10 mm in size and classified as EU-TIRADS 5
- Nodules > 15 mm in size and classified as EU-TIRADS 4 or 5
- Nodules > 20 mm in size and classified as EU-TIRADS 3 to 5
- Nodules > 20 mm in size and classified as EU-TIRADS 2 if they are compressives
- Nodules < 10 mm in size and classified as EU-TIRADS 5 can either be punctured or closely monitored.
- Presence of suspicious lymph nodes

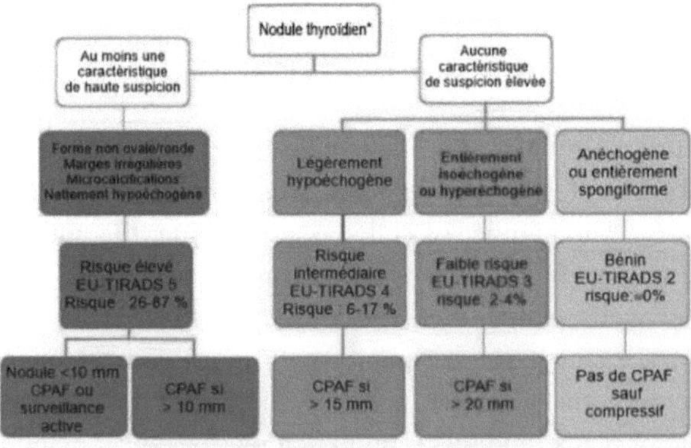

Figure 1: EU-TIRADS algorithm for risk stratification of malignancyand the indication for cytopuncture of the thyroid nodule [21].

In its latest recommendations (2015) [19], the American Thyroid Association (ATA) proposes a strategy for evaluating thyroid nodules based on levels of ultrasound suspicion of malignancy, on the one hand, and on nodule size, on the other (Table II).

Table II: Indications for CPAF according to the 2015 ATA recommendations [19].

Level of suspicion of malignancy	Ultrasound characteristics	Estimated risk of malignancy	CPAF/size threshold (largest dimension)
High suspicion	Solid hyperechoic nodule or solid hypoechoic component of a partially cystic nodule with one or more of the following characteristics: irregular boundaries (infiltrative, microlobulated), microcalcifications, shape thicker than wide, annular calcifications. with a tissue component, proven extra-thyroidal extension	70-90 %	Recommended if size of nodule ≥ 01 cm
Intermediate suspicion	Hypoechoic solid nodule with regular margins free of microcalcifications/extra thyroidal extensions/thicker than normal shape large	10-20 %	Recommended if size of nodule ≥ 01 cm
Low suspicion	Isoechoic or hyperechoic solid nodule, or partially cystic nodule with eccentric solid areas without microcalcifications/irregular margins/extra-thyroidal extension/thicker than normal shape. large	5-10 %	Recommended if size of nodule ≥ 1.5 cm
Very low suspicion	Spongiform or partially spongiform nodules without any of the ultrasound characteristics described in the low/intermediate/high suspicion profiles	< 3 %	Recommended if nodule size ≥ 02 cm, observation without CPAF is also a reasonable option
Benign nodules	Purely cystic nodules (no solid component)	< 1 %	No CPAF (aspiration of the cyst may be considered for symptomatic drainage, or cosmetics)

ATA states in its latest publication in 2022 that the decision to perform CPAF should be based on individual risk stratification with reference to the patient's history and clinical and ultrasound data. Nodules less than 1cm in size should be punctured if there is more than one ultrasound feature of malignancy, cervical lymphadenopathy or a high-risk history; otherwise, solid nodules greater than 1cm with only one ultrasound feature of malignancy should be punctured [9] (Table III).

Table III: Indications for CPAF according to the ATA 2022 recommendations [9].

Clinical features and/or ultrasound of the thyroid nodule	Recommended size threshold for CPAF	
History of high risk		
Nodule with characteristics ultrasound examination of suspected malignancy	> 5mm	Recommendation A
Nodule with no ultrasound features suspicion of malignancy	> 5mm	Recommendation I
Abnormal cervical lymph nodes	All	Recommendation A
Microcalcifications in the nodule	>= 1 cm	Recommendation B
Solid nodule		
Hypoechoic	>= 1 cm	Recommendation B
Iso or hyperechoic	>= 1-1.5 cm Recommendation C	
Mixed cystic-solid nodule		
With any feature ultrasound investigation of suspected malignancy	>= 1.5-2 cm Recommendation B	
Without ultrasound characteristics of suspected malignancy	>= 2 cm	Recommendation C
	>= 2 cm	Recommendation C
Spongiform nodule	(ultrasound monitoring without	
	puncture can be an alternative	
	acceptable	
Purely cystic nodule	CPAF not indicated (except for symptomatic or cosmetic drainage) Recommendation E	

Explanation of recommendations : A, strong recommendation based on solid evidence; B, recommendation based on fair evidence; C, recommendation based on expert opinion; E, recommendation not recommended based on fair evidence; I, recommends neither for nor against due to lack of evidence. With regard to multinodular goitres, in its 2015 recommendations, ATA recommends puncturing nodules >= 01 cm or larger that are sonographically suspicious and the largest nodules, >= 02 cm regardless of their sonographic characteristics.

1.5 Benefits

Ultrasound-guided CPAF is the most useful and reliable method for assessing thyroid nodules [22]. It is a simple, rapid, painless and reproducible technique [23] that can be performed on an outpatient basis, without fasting and without local anaesthetic. Its main objective is to reduce the frequency of surgery for thyroid nodules [24].At present, CPAF is considered to be the "gold standard" for exploring thyroid nodules [25].

1.6 Effects

Major complications of CPAF are extremely rare [26]; minor pain persisting for more than 24 hours, vagal discomfort or haematomas may occur, but these side-effects are not serious and are spontaneously reversible.According to the experience of the Gharib Hossein and John Goellner team, who performed more than 11,000 thyroid punctures over 12 years, there were no major haemorrhagic complications, even in patients taking salicylates or anticoagulants. surgical excision one day after aspiration [27].

Rarely, during puncture, the trachea may be perforated or there may be damage to the recurrent nerve, which is reversible. Necrosis of the nodule after cytopuncture, due to interruption of the microcirculation, is rare but does occur; it can be seen especially in a malignant nodule and in less than two weeks [28].

The risk of tumour spread is extremely rare with fine needle aspiration and only a few individual cases have been reported and tumour spread is usually associated with highly malignant anaplastic carcinoma [29]. However, intra-glandular haemorrhage, follicular destruction, fibrosis, granulation tissue formation, nuclear or cellular atypia and capsular changes may occur, and these are rare side-effects. Finally, a retrospective Japanese study carried out in 1992 on 500 thyroid cytoponctions revealed transient post-puncture hyperthyroidism (within 02 to 20 days) in 5 cases. The explanation for this hyperthyroidism is not known, but several authors suggest the occurrence of post-puncture inflammatory phenomena leading to the release of thyroid hormones.

1.7 Limits

The two main disadvantages of CPAF are false-negative cytology and failure to detect microcarcinomas, either through misinterpretation or, more often, inadequate sampling [30, 31].

Although CPAF can establish a diagnosis of papillary carcinoma based mainly on cytological features [32], it is considered uninterpretable in 10 to 20% of cases, which generally correspond to cystic lesions and inadequate sampling, or simply "suspicious" in 9 to 38% of cases and mainly concerns vesicular tumours (oncocytic) and microvesicular tumours whose malignant nature cannot be determined by cytology [33, 34, 35].

CPAF is also unable to distinguish between adenoma and vesicular carcinoma as analysis of vascular and capsular invasion of the thyroid gland requires a full histological examination [32].

1.8 Result : Examination cytology

Bethesda system for Reporting Thyroid Cytopathology establishes a standardised reporting system with a limited number of diagnostic categories for CPAF. Using this classification, cytopathologists can communicate their interpretations to the clinician in succinct, unambiguous and clinically useful terms [36, 37].

The Bethesda classification is widely adopted in the European Union and in many parts of the world and is endorsed and recommended by ATA [38]. This system improves communication and provides a uniform model for sharing data among investigators. However, since its acceptance in clinical practice, questions have arisen about the appropriate use of diagnostic categories, the associated risks of malignancy and appropriate management. Revisions are made and currently reference is made to the 2017 revision inspired by new data and new developments in the field of thyroid pathology. Guidelines have been revised for the management of patients with thyroid nodules, such as the introduction of molecular tests to complement cytopathological examination and the reclassification of the non-invasive follicular variant of papillary thyroid carcinoma as "thyroid nodule". NIFT-P. Thus, thyroid cytology results provide six main diagnostic categories:

1.8.1Bethesda classification (Appendix III)

1.8.1.1 Bethesda I: Category "non-diagnostic" (ND) or "unsatisfactory" (UNS)

This category includes unsatisfactory cytological specimens for which a cytological opinion is not possible. Examples include specimens with profuse haemorrhage, poor cell preservation and an insufficient sample of follicular cells.A sample is considered satisfactory for evaluation if it contains at least 06 groups of well visualised follicular cells (well fixed, well stained and undistorted), each group must be composed of at least 10 cells. Given that the vast majority of ND/UNS nodules turn out to be benign, reducing the number of follicular cells required for diagnosis would spare many patients repeated CPAF and significantly reduce ND/UNS findings without significantly impacting on the false-negative rate [39, 40].In this context, the 2017 version of the Bethesda system brings several advantages exceptions to the follicular cell count requirement :

- Any specimen that contains abundant colloid is suitable for evaluation even if 06 groups of follicular cells are not identified; a poorly cellular specimen with abundant colloid is implicitly a predominantly macrofollicular nodule and therefore certainly benign.

- Whenever a specific diagnosis (e.g. lymphocytic thyroiditis) can be made, as long as there are no significant cellular atypia, the specimen is considered adequate for evaluation.

Specimens consisting solely of cystic content (macrophages) are considered ND/UNS; their significance and clinical value depend largely on ultrasound correlation. Cytologies classified in this category vary from 1.8% to 23.6% depending on the series in the literature [91], but should ideally be limited to 10% of cases. Repeated puncture with ultrasound guidance is recommended for nodules classified as ND/UNS after 03 months [41]; it is diagnostic in most cases, but some nodules persist as ND/UNS, in which case surgical removal is envisaged.

1.8.1.2 Bethesda II: "benign" category (Figure 2)

This second category of the Bethesda system groups together benign cytologies and is encountered in 60% of thyroid cytologies. [42]; it is characterised by variable amounts of colloid, benign-appearing follicular (or vesicular) cells, oncocytic (hurthle) cells and macrophages. This category includes:

• All thyroiditis (most often lymphocytic or Hashimoto's thyroiditis) is interpreted as benign.

• Benign lesions with similar cytological characteristics are classified histologically as nodular goitre, colloid nodules, hyperplastic nodules, vesicular adenomas and nodules in Graves' disease. Cytological study does not allow differentiation between these entities. histology, but this does not alter the management, which is conservative.

Benign vesicular nodules have the following diagnostic criteria: sparsely to moderately cellular specimen, cells often regularly arranged in monostratified flaps, small (haematoid-sized) basophilic nuclei, more or less abundant colloid substance of variable consistency, few microvesicles, histiocytes frequently present and often pigmented and/or fibroblasts, inflammatory cells if thyroiditis. Monitoring of the nodule over a period of 3 to 5 years is recommended, with an initial ultrasound check in 6 to 18 months; if the nodule has changed little or not at all, monitoring should continue within this timeframe. A second puncture is not recommended unless there have been significant radiological changes. If the nodule increases in size or if any ultrasound features suspicious of malignancy appear, surgical removal of the nodule is considered.

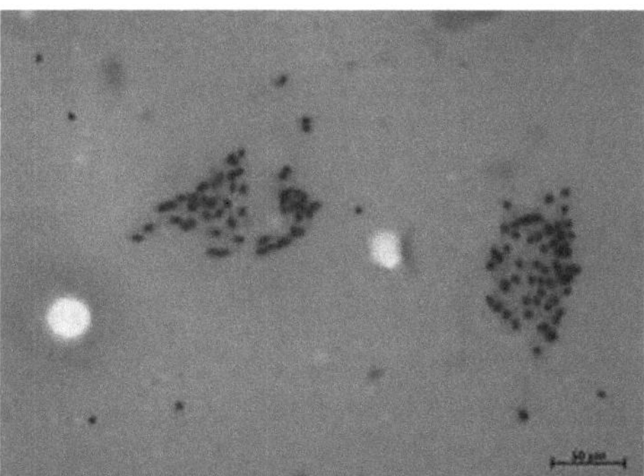

Figure 1: benign cytology (HEX200)

1.8.1.3 Bethesda III: Category "follicular lesion of undetermined significance" or "atypia of undetermined significance" (FSU/FLUS) (Figure 3).

This category includes thyroid cytologies containing cells with architectural and/or nuclear atypia. These atypia are insufficient to be classified as "malignant" or "malignant".One part is "suspicious of malignancy" and the other part is large enough to be classified as "malignant"."benign". Bethesda's latest version of 2017 recommends the sub-classification of atypia, even if this does not affect patient management:

i. Cytological atypia: can take several forms: focal nuclear changes, mild but widespread nuclear atypia, atypical cystic epithelial coating, or "histiocytoid" cells [43, 44].

ii. Architectural atypia: this is often a specimen that is not very cellular, but composed mainly of microfollicles.

iii. Cytological and architectural atypia: cytological atypia and architectural atypicalities.

iv. Oncocytic (Hurthle) cells AUS/FLUS: this is often a poorly cellular sample composed exclusively of Hurthle cells or predominantly of Hurthle cells if the clinical context strongly suggests a benign Hurthle cell nodule (lymphocytic thyroiditis or a GMN).

v. Non-specific type atypia (NOS).

This category requires repeat ultrasound-guided CPAF within 3 to 6 months, and if the diagnosis of AUS/FLUS persists, surgical excision is recommended (table IV).The rate of cytology classified as III AUS/FLUS varies between 1% and 18% depending on the series in the literature. This category should be considered as a category of last resort. In fact, the Bethesda system recommends making an effort to limit its use to around 7% of all CPAF results. This is proving a difficult challenge for many laboratories, and a more realistic limit would be 10% [98, 99].

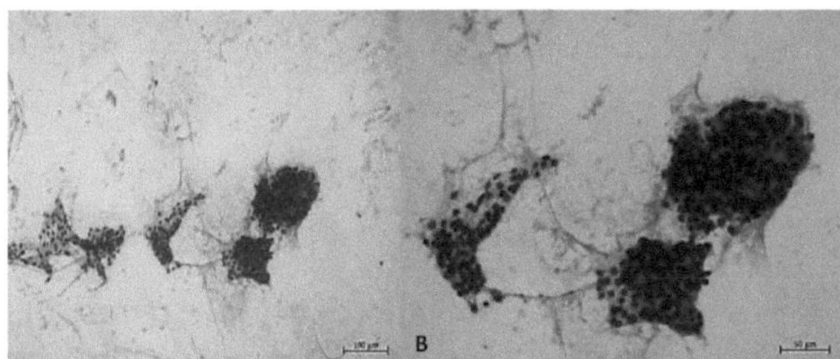

Figure 3: Bethesda III: cytology in favour of a follicular lesion of undetermined significance A(HEx100); B(HEx200)

1.8.1.4 Bethesda IV: Follicular neoplasm or suspected follicular neoplasm (FN and SFN) (Figure 4)

Some laboratories prefer SFN because a significant proportion of cases (up to 35%) turn out not to be neoplasms but rather hypertrophic proliferations of follicular cells, often seen in cases of GMN [45, 46]. The Bethesda 2017 system makes a change to the definition and diagnostic criteria for this category in light of NIFT-P.Initially, cases showing the nuclear features of papillary thyroid carcinoma were excluded from this category. In the new 2017 version, cases with follicular or vesicular architecture with mild nuclear changes (increased nuclear size, nuclear contour irregularity and/or chromatin compensation) can be classified in this category as long as true papillae and intranuclear pseudoinclusions are absent [47]. The presence of architectural features suggestive of a follicular neoplasm, together with the nuclear features cited above, raise the possibility of an invasive follicular variant of papillary carcinoma (FVPTC) or its indolent counterpart NIFT-P. Definitive distinction between these entities is not possible on cytological material.In their meta-analysis, Bongiovanni et al [101] found a wide range of percentages of cases classified in this category in relation to all cases in the different studies, from 1.2 to 25.3%, with an average of 10.1%. The recommended treatment for FN/SFN is surgical excision, which will is most often a lobectomy.

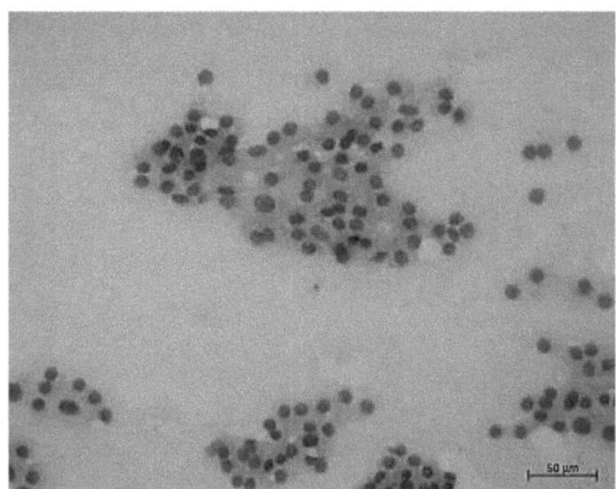

Figure 4: Follicular neoplasm on cytology (HEx200)

1.8.1.5 Bethesda V: Category suspected of malignancy

This fifth category covers cytologies showing cells with cytonuclear abnormalities, but malignancy cannot be confirmed, either because the number of cells is insufficient, or because one or two criteria are missing to allow a formal diagnosis.This category includes the different types of cancer as well as NIFT-P. In each case, it is necessary to specify the type of cancer suspected (papillary carcinoma, medullary carcinoma, differentiated carcinoma, anaplastic carcinoma, lymphoma or metastasis). Surgical removal should be the preferred treatment [42].

1.8.1.6 Bethesda VI: 'Clever' category (Figure 5)

This category is used whenever the cytomorphological features are conclusive of malignancy. The new 2017 Bethesda version changes the definition and criteria for papillary thyroid carcinoma cases to avoid false positives due to NIFT-P. It recommends limiting the use of the "malignant" category to cases presenting "classic" characteristics of papillary thyroid carcinoma (true papillae, psammomatous bodies and nuclear pseudo-inclusions) [50,51]. Despite these limitations, a small proportion of cases (3 to 4%) diagnosed as malignant are subsequently found to be NIFT-P on definitive histopathological examination. Surgical removal should be the preferred treatment (Table IV).

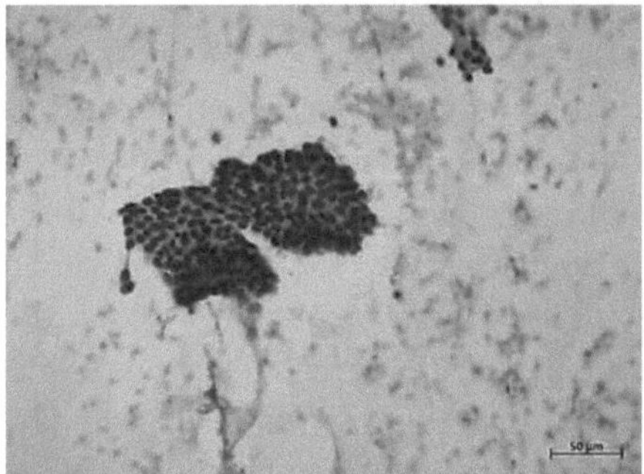

Figure 5: cytology in favour of papillary carcinoma (HEx200)

Table IV: Risk of malignancy and action to be taken for each category of the 2017 Bethesda classification

Tableau. Système de Bethesda.		
Catégories cytologiques	**Risque de malignité (%)**	**Conduite à tenir proposée**
I - Non diagnostique	1-4	2e cytoponction échoguidée à 3 mois
II - Bénin	0-3	Surveillance échographique
III - Atypies de signification indéterminée (ASI)/ lésion folliculaire de signification indéterminée (LFSI)	5 -15	2e cytoponction échoguidée à 3-6 mois
IV - Néoplasme folliculaire (NF) Néoplasme folliculaire à cellules oncocytaires (NFO)	15-30	Chirurgie (lobectomie)
V - Suspect de malignité	60-75	Chirurgie (thyroïdectomie ou lobectomie)
VI - Malin (type de cancer suspecté à préciser)	97-99	Chirurgie (thyroïdectomie)

1.9 Other methods associated

1.9.1 Immunocytochemistry

1.9.1.1 Detection of thyroglobulin

Thyroglobulin is easily detected, but its intensity varies according to the histological type of lesion: very high immunoreactivity for differentiated vesicular carcinomas and their metastases (95-100%), lower immunoreactivity for microvesicular, trabecular or papillary carcinomas (61-100%) and negative or weakly positive immunoreactivity for anaplastic carcinomas (15-50%). Its detection on cytopsy slides makes it possible to confirm the primary thyroid nature of a lesion and to make the differential diagnosis of a metastasis, which is very useful in the case of revealing metastases without an obvious thyroid tumour and for certain primary tumours that are difficult to interpret anatomopathologically [52].

1.9.1.2 Detection of Calcitonin

Calcitonin detection is used to diagnose medullary thyroid carcinoma (MTC) and to differentiate it from undifferentiated and anaplastic carcinomas [53]. In addition to its therapeutic value, this diagnosis is even more important in the case of familial forms.

1.9.2 Molecular biology

In vesicular carcinoma, the PAX8-PPAR gamma chromosomal rearrangement is fairly constant. This rearrangement is not found in papillary carcinomas. However, it should be noted that 10-30% of vesicular adenomas also present these genetic anomalies [57].

Two types of molecular alteration are described for papillary carcinomas [58]:

• Epigenetic anomalies: these are overexpressions of c-Met and of EGFR [59].

• Structural genetic abnormalities: RET/PTC and TRK rearrangements and BRAF mutations [59, 60].

The Ras mutation is more frequently detected in vesicular variants of papillary carcinoma than in classic papillary carcinoma [59, 63].

1.9.3Quantitative cytology: quantification of DNA

This technique is proposed in selected cases, in particular in cases of doubtful cytology and especially for follicular neoplasms.This technique, based on the quantitative study of nuclear DNA, is performed on a fresh, unfixed material with excellent cellular material or on cytobloc. It makes it possible to determine the DNA index (which is the ratio between the DNA content of the cells studied and the control cells) and the distribution of the cells in the cell cycle, thus obtaining histograms which may correspond to diploidy (normal DNA content), aneuploidy (abnormal DNA content) or polyploidy (increased DNA content). Results are variable and several authors suggest that quantitative cytology has limited diagnostic value [64].

2 EXTEMPORANEOUS EXAMINATION (EE)

The development of cytopuncture and its recent standardisation has had a negative impact on the role of EE in thyroid pathology, which has gone from being the predominant examination in thyroid surgery to an ancillary examination. Indeed, the additional contribution of EE is questioned by surgeons on the one hand, and by cytopathologists on the other, who are confronted with erroneous results due to problems of orientation, unfixed samples, freezing artefacts and poorly visible nuclear details [67].EE is a highly specific examination with a specificity of 100%, but not very sensitive, with a sensitivity of between 50 and 92%. Sensitivity depends on the histological type, and is low for vesicular carcinoma (varying from 8 to 36%) since examination of the entire capsule to detect capsular effraction or vascular invasion cannot be performed until the definitive histological examination [68]. Most authors recommend EE only in the case of suspicious or uncertain cytopuncture, to guide surgical extension in cases confirmed as malignant, or if unexpected lesions are found during surgery [68].

3 ANATOMOPATHOLOGICAL STUDY

Thyroid cancer is one of the most common endocrine tumours in the world, accounting for around 1% of all cancers, hence the importance of anatomopathological examination, which should be carried out systematically on any surgical excision specimen to enable a definitive distinction to be made between a benign lesion and a malignant one, and to detect other nodules that may escape clinical examination and paraclinical investigations.

In 2017, the WHO established a new classification of thyroid tumours that makes corrections to follicular tumours (Appendix IV) [31].

3.1 Benign thyroid nodules

3.1.1Vesicular adenoma (Figure 6)

This is the most common cause of thyroid nodules. It is a benign tumour with signs of vesicular differentiation and no capsular or vascular invasion.

***Macroscopic appearance:** the nodule is solid or cystic, fleshy or colloid, light brown in colour. It is well limited, often encapsulated and of variable size (from 1 to 10 cm).

***Microscopic appearance:**

- The capsule is thin and regular, well limited and without signs of invasion. vascular or capsular.
- Cellularity is variable, the nuclei are regular in size and shape, the nucleoli are inconspicuous, the cytoplasm is eosinophilic, clear or amphophilic and the stroma is small, well vascularised and may contain degenerative changes.
- Depending on the type of vesicle and supporting stroma, there are microvesicular, normovesicular, macrovesicular and trabecular adenomas.

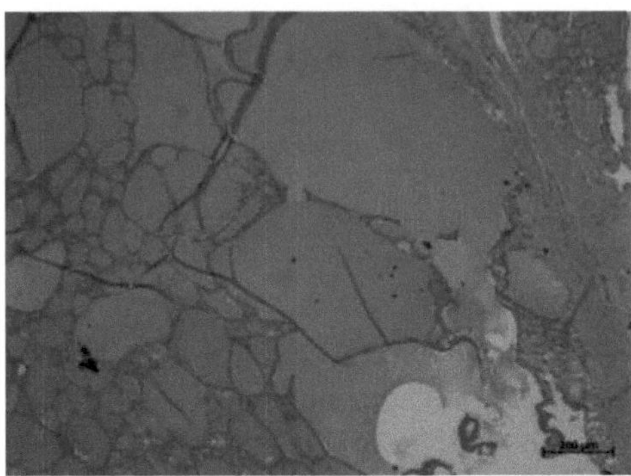

Figure 6: Benign vesicular adenoma on definitive histological examination (HEx 50)

3.1.2Oncocytic adenoma (Hurthle) [69] (Figure 7)

Oncocytic adenoma is a fairly rare benign tumour accounting for 20% of cases. benign thyroid tumours. Macroscopically, the tumour is often >=2 cm in size, solitary, fleshy, light brown to mahogany in colour, lobulated and surrounded by a capsule of variable thickness. Microscopically, it is made up of at least 75% oncocytic cells with an often follicular, more rarely trabecular, architecture. Oncocytic cells are large, sharply outlined cells with abundant, highly eosinophilic, granular cytoplasm. They have a large pleomorphic nucleus centred by a prominent nucleolus. The nucleus is sometimes wrinkled or indented. These atypia are common but are not synonymous with malignancy.

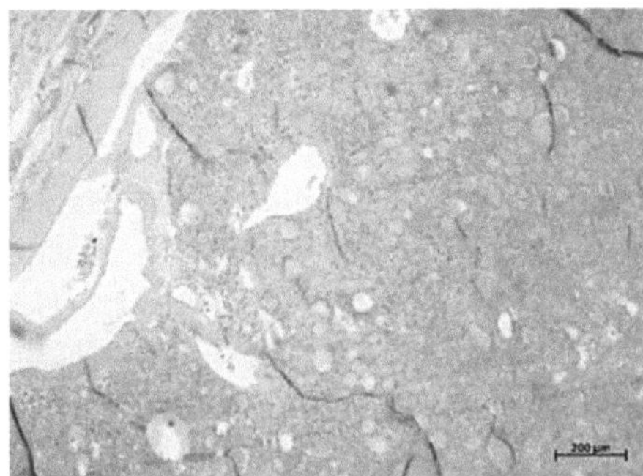

Figure 7: Benign oncocytic adenoma (HEx50)

3.2 Other vesicular thyroid tumours encapsulated

This category corresponds to a group of encapsulated vesicular thyroid tumours of uncertain malignancy, the most frequent ofwhich is (Figure8)
As recommended by the National Cancer Institute in 2012 [70], a review of follicular thyroid neoplasms characterised by low clinical risk has been carried out. As a result, a revision of the nomenclature has been proposed in order to reduce overtreatment of certain thyroid nodules and thus reduce the psychological and clinical consequences associated with a cancer diagnosis [70]. In particular, follicular variant papillary thyroid carcinoma (FVPTC) accounts for 30% of carcinomas and includes encapsulated, invasive encapsulated and non-encapsulated forms [71]. A thorough re-evaluation of non-invasive encapsulated and invasive encapsulated forms by international experts was completed in 2016 with the publication that proposed the introduction of NIFT-P (Non Invasive Follicular neoplasm with Papillary-like nuclear features) [72]. The results of the study showed that non-invasive encapsulated forms of FVPTC with specific histological features have extremely indolent behaviour and no adverse events in 109 patients followed for 13 years. These experts defined very precise histological criteria to define these lesions:

*Macroscopic criteria: the nodule is variable in size (from one to several centimetres), usually beige in colour, firm in consistency, encapsulated and well circumscribed.

*Microscopic criteria: according to the strict histological criteria for inclusion and exclusion [71], NIFT-P is an encapsulated or clearly demarcated papillary cancer with predominant follicles and the nuclear characteristics of papillary thyroid carcinoma. The first important criterion is therefore the demonstration of complete encapsulation of the lesion. The presence of papillary-type nuclear changes must be noted according to:

- size and shape (nuclear enlargement, overlap and/or elongation),

-irregularities in the nuclear membrane (furrows with irregular contours and/or pseudo-inclusions)

-chromatin characteristics (chromatin margination at the membrane and/or glassy nuclei).

For each class of these nuclear characteristics, a score of 0 or 1 is assigned, giving a score between 0 and 3. For the diagnosis of NIFT-P, a nuclear score between 2 and 3 is required. Furthermore, according to the diagnostic criteria initially proposed [72], the diagnosis of NIFT-P cannot be made if any of the following exclusion criteria are present: vascular or capsular invasion, more than 1% papillae, presence of psammoma bodies, more than 30% solid trabecular architecture. However, a refinement of the diagnostic criteria was proposed in 2018 [73]: the 1% papillae threshold has been modified, and in the presence of true papillae the lesion cannot be considered as NIFT-P. Indeed, it has been shown that the presence of papillae (even in less than 1% of tumour areas) is associated with a higher frequency of BRAFV600E mutation and metastatic lymph node occurrence [74, 75], compared to NIFT-P with total absence of papillae. Another change is that in the case of a nuclear score of 3, which reflects a pronounced expression of the nuclear characteristics of papillary carcinoma, a careful revision of the entire tumour is recommended to exclude the presence of papillae [73]. These cases were considered benign since NIFT-Ps have a good prognosis regardless of nodule size [76] and can be managed by thyroid lobectomy as for patients with benign thyroid neoplasms [77].

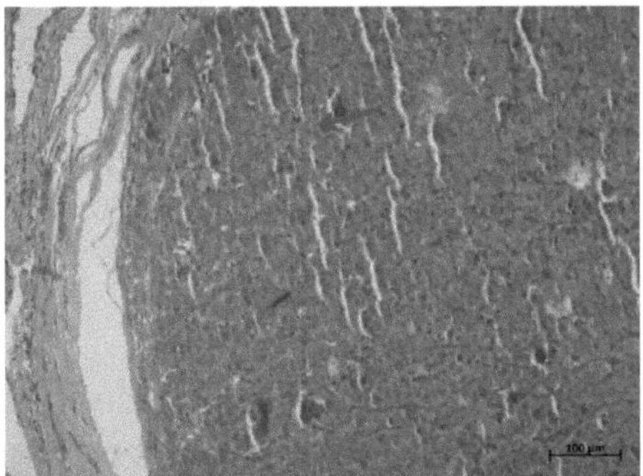

Figure 8: GMN with discovery of NIFT-P and microcarcinoma papillary 0.1 cm on definitive examination (HEx100)

3.3 Malignant thyroid nodules

They are represented by thyroid carcinomas in 99% of cases, which develop from thyreocytes in 90% of cases and more rarely from C cells. Non-carcinomatous tumours (which do not arise from epithelial cells) are mainly lymphomas and sarcomas of the intervesicular connective tissue. There are also secondary tumours or metastases, which are rare. We will detail the characteristics of certain thyroid carcinomas found in our results.

3.3.1Papillary carcinoma (PC) [78] (Figure 9)

Thyroid prostate cancer is a differentiated cancer of follicular origin and accounts for around 90% of thyroid carcinomas.

***Macroscopic appearance**: PC can be solid or cystic with papillary growths in the classic variant. Solid PCs are often beige in colour and firm in consistency. They are often multifocal but may be encapsulated or infiltrate the adjacent thyroid parenchyma.

***Microscopic appearance**: the CP is formed by

- Branched, complex papillae with random orientation and vesicles
- Follicular cells have pathognomonic nuclear features: overlapping nuclei with clear, finely dispersed chromatin giving a ground-glass appearance, eosinophilic intranuclear inclusions and longitudinal nuclear grooves giving a coffee-bean appearance.
- Abundant stroma with dense fibrosis giving a star-like appearance. Elastosis of the stroma is found in 2/3 of cases [79].
- Psammomas can be found in the fibrous stroma of prostate cancer.

(rounded, onion-bubble calcifications) in half the cases.

- Note that when the vesicular architecture is exclusive, we speak of CP

vesicular architecture.

***Immunohistochemistry:** PCs express specific antibodies: Tg, galectin-3, HBME-1 and TTF-1.

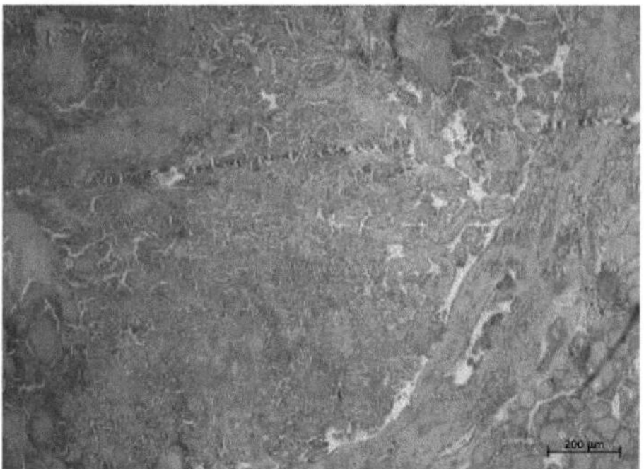

Figure 9: Papillary carcinoma on definitive histological examination (HEx50)

3.3.2 Vesicular carcinoma (VC) [80, 81] (Figure 10)

CV is a follicular differentiated carcinoma without nuclei with the characteristics of prostate cancer, with invasion of the thyroid parenchyma (non-encapsulated invasive form) or capsular invasion and/or angioinvasion (encapsulated form).

CVs are less lymphophilic than PCs, which give rise to more lymph node metastases, but they give rise to more distant metastases (especially bone, lung or liver) through vascular extension.

***Macroscopic appearance:** the CV is often single, of variable size (from one to several cm), rounded, pinkish-beige in colour, fleshy with some cystic or haemorrhagic changes. It is surrounded by a thick, irregular capsule which distinguishes it from an adenoma.

***Microscopic appearance:** the nodule contains vesicles surrounded by thyreocytes with rounded, fairly regular nuclei; the following criteria are used to diagnose malignancy:

- Complete capsular breach in shirt button
- Vascular invasion of a capsular vessel or beyond, the tumour cell sheet in the vascular lumen must be covered by endothelial cells or associated with a thrombus.

CV sometimes poses a problem of differential diagnosis with vesicular adenoma, as the nuclear abnormalities are discrete and uncharacteristic and capsular effusion is sometimes difficult to detect.

For this reason, the diagnosis of CV requires a complete sampling of the capsule and often several levels of sections on the same sample when capsular effraction is suspected. This sampling is only possible during the definitive anatomopathological examination.

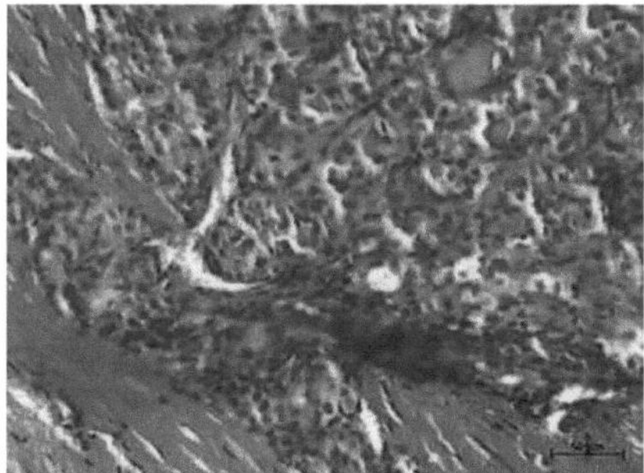

Figure 10: Vesicular carcinoma with minimal capsular invasion (HEx200)

3.3.3Poorly differentiated carcinoma

Poorly differentiated carcinoma is often difficult to diagnose because the histological appearance is often polymorphic with a more differentiated contingent; it includes insular cancers with a trabecular contingent, and certain papillary cancers with tall or cylindrical cells and a trabecular contingent; it is often large with invasion of the thyroid capsule, lymph node metastases and distant metastases, and its prognosis is more serious.

3.3.4 Medullary carcinoma (MC) [82] (Figure 11)

CM is a rare tumour which develops on the C cells responsible for secreting calcitonin.

***Macroscopic appearance:** the nodule is generally whitish, well-defined, not visible to the naked eye. encapsulated and often located at the upper-middle third union.

***Microscopic appearance:**

- Tumour cells have a granular cytoplasm and uniform round or oval nuclei with granular chromatin, together giving the "salt and pepper" appearance characteristic of endocrine tumours.
- The stroma is dense with amyloid calcitonin deposits, prominent vascularisation and calcifications.

***Immunohistochemistry:** CMT shows positive immunostaining for calcitonin in over 80% of cases.

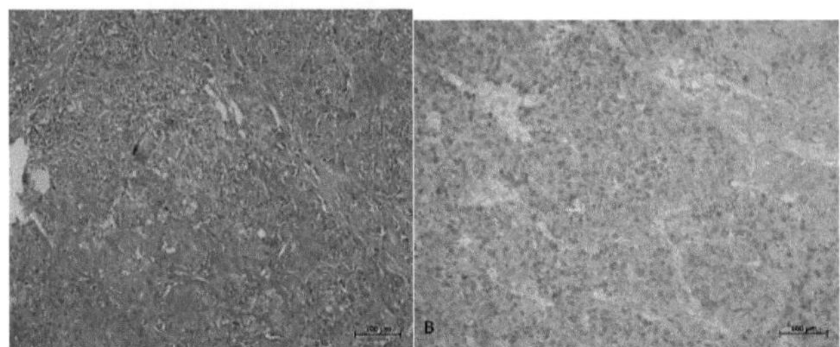

Figure 11: CASE 1: A) histological appearance of medullary carcinoma (HEx100); B) positive for calcitonin x100.

3.3.5 Thyroid metastases

The primary tumours most likely to give rise to thyroid metastasis are: lung cancer, breast cancer (Figure 12), oesophageal cancer, renal cell carcinoma, melanoma and gynaecological cancers [83].Thyroid metastases generally have the same histological and immunohistochemical characteristics as the primary tumour.

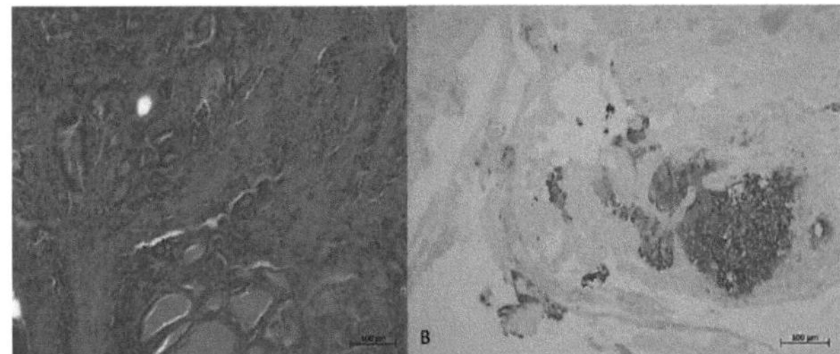

Figure 122: CASE 2: A) Histological appearance of a thyroid metastasis of mammary origin (star) note the presence of adjacent thyroid vesicles (arrow) (HEx100); B) Her2 positive at 3+ (x100).

4 CYTOHISTOLOGICAL CORRELATION

In the literature, the figures on the performance of the CPAF in the exploration of thyroid nodules vary from study to study. Interpretation of these data is tricky due to the variability of the classifications used and the methods employed in the statistical analyses, as well as other biases (the heterogeneous nature of the samples studied and the absence of histological control of all the nodules punctured) [84, 85].

Bongiovanni et al [86], in their metanalysis published in 2012, when they considered category III as a positive sample in the statistical analysis, they found that the sensitivity of CPAF did not change much (from 97% to 97.2%) and the PPV decreased slightly (from 55.9% to 46.9%) [86].

A meta-analysis published in 2012 in which Massimo Bongiovanni et al [87] compiled the results of 8 studies involving 25445 patients who had undergone CPAF, 6362 of whom had undergone surgery, the results of the cytohistological correlation study gave a sensitivity of 97%, a specificity of 50.1%, a PPV of 55.9% and an NPV of 96.3%. A Brazilian study was published in 2018 in the European Thyroid Journal in which Reuters K.B. et al [88] studied a series of 585 patients followed for thyroid nodules at the São Paulo Thyroid Disease Centre, 980 CPAFs were performed and 245 patients underwent surgery over a 2-year period. Analysis of the cyto-histological correlation gave a sensitivity of 92.1%, a specificity of 67.8%, a PPV of 61.4% and an NPV of 93.9%.A study published in 2015 and carried out by Hajmanoechehri et al [89] who studied 101 cases of patients with thyroid nodules who had received CPAF and The results of the cyto-histological correlation analysis gave a sensitivity of 95.2%, a specificity of 68.4%, a PPV of 83.3% and an NPV of 89.6%. In the same framework, Muratli et al [90] published in 2014 a series of 1333 patients with CPAF, they found a sensitivity of 87.1%, a specificity of 64.6%, a PPV of 76.1% and an NPV of 79.5%. In a study published in 2020 of 100 patients with thyroid nodules who had undergone CPAF and undergone surgery at the Pondicherry Institute of Medical Sciences in India, Anand B et al [91] found a sensitivity of 72.4%, a specificity of 94.3%, a PPV of 84% and an NPV of 89.2%.Seiberling et al [92], in their retrospective study carried out between September 2005 and February 2007 and including 203 patients followed for thyroid nodules, reported a sensitivity of 100%, a specificity of 73%, a PPV of 57.1% and an NPV of 100%. (Table V)

Table V: Sensitivity, specificity, PPV and NPV of cytology in different series

Series	Sensitivity	Specific	VPP	VPN
Bongiovanni et al [87].	97%	50,1%	55,9%	96,3%
Reuters K.B. et al [88]	92,1%	67,8%	61,4%	93,9%
Hajmanoechehri et al [89].	95,2%	68,4%	83,3%	89,6%
Muratli et al [90]	87,1%	64,6%	76,1%	79,5%
Anand B. et al [91]	72,4%	94,3%	84%	89,2%
Seiberling et al [92]	100%	73%	57,1%	100%

Other studies report higher rates of sensitivity and specificity, which is linked to the exclusion of some or all undetermined or suspicious cases (i.e. specimens classified as "AUS/FLUS", "FN/SFN" and suspected of malignancy) from the statistical calculation [93, 94], which leads to a reduction in the number of reported false positives and false negatives and therefore an exaggeration of the accuracy of CPAF [95]. The Bethesda system has made a crucial contribution to the investigation of thyroid nodules by classifying the results of CPAFs into 6 cytological categories, leading to the standardisation of thyroid cytology investigation. Each of these categories may be associated with an implicit risk of malignancy, resulting in a recommendation for the management of thyroid nodules [96].

4. 1 Bethesda I category

The risk of malignancy for the "ND/UNS" category is difficult to calculate since most nodules in this category are not resected. Among nodules reported as "ND/UNS" and operated on, the rate of malignancy is 9 to 32% but this value overestimates malignant tumours compared with the cohort as a whole since operated nodules are only a selected subset which have worrying clinical and/or ultrasound characteristics or which are repeatedly "ND/UNS"; a reasonable extrapolation of the risk of malignancy is 5 to 10% [40] (Table VI). The rate of malignancy in this category is difficult to assess as only a small subset of nodules classified as "ND/UNS" undergo surgical resection, so there is a disparity in the rate of malignancy between different studies, ranging from 0% to 63.2% [98, 99]. Ultrasound-guided CPAF for small nodules and nodules that are heterogeneous on palpation provides aspiration from the exact pathological site and thus reduces cytologies in this category; in addition, operator experience plays a crucial role in limiting specimens in this category [26].

4. 2 Bethesda II category

According to the Bethesda system, the "benign" category is associated with a low risk of malignancy of 0 to 3% [100]. The false-negative rate varies between 0% and 6.9% (table VI). In this context, it should be noted that cystic remodelling can occur in neoplastic lesions in the thyroid gland, making it difficult to sample the solid part of the tumour and, in turn, miss malignancy [102, 103, 104]. Many factors can contribute to the diagnosis of false negatives: a study of the factors leading to the diagnosis of false negatives has shown that there is a positive correlation between the size of thyroid nodules and the rate of cases diagnosed as false negatives [102].

4. 3 Bethesda III category

The rate of malignancy in category III "AUS/FLUS" varies between 5% and 15% [105], and can reach 50% in certain series in the literature [89]. Measurement of the elasticity of thyroid nodules using the elastography technique may have a place in these doubtful cases, but prospective evaluation studies are still needed. Current management now includes the use of molecular tests.

4. 4 Bethesda IV category

For nodules classified as Bethesda IV, the percentage of malignancy in the literature varies from 5.7 to 37 % [89,106] (table VI). These two cases of malignant thyroid tumours were a papillary carcinoma and a medullary carcinoma on definitive histological study; this raises the question of why they were not classified in category V "suspected of malignancy", For the papillary carcinoma, one explanation is that the sampling only involved the vesicular structures of the papillary carcinoma. Indeed, in the absence of true papillary structures, differentiation of papillary carcinoma from follicular neoplasm may be difficult because nuclear changes in papillary carcinoma may be slight or focal, and also because cytological features such as nuclear furrows may be seen in other lesions, particularly in low cell smears [107]. Schreiner et al [108] found that adenomatoid nodules were the main cause of poor cytohistological correlation in follicular neoplasms. Agglutination and crowding of follicular cells may be observed if aspiration is performed on a hyperplastic thyroid nodule and give architectural atypia [104].Useful criteria for differentiating nodular goitre from follicular adenoma include higher cellularity, uniform cellularity, uniform nuclear enlargement, syncytial clusters, predominant micro follicles and sparse colloid [103]. A further point to note is that, as with Pandey et al [103] and Yang et al [109], we have found that over-emphasis on the presence of micro follicular structures or clumped cells in poor quality samples can lead to a false positive diagnosis. Molecular tests can be used to further assess the risk of malignancy rather than proceeding directly to surgery.

4. 5 Bethesda V category

For category V "suspected malignancy", the malignancy rate varies from 60 to 100% according to the different series in the literature [106, 110]. The presence of false positive cases may be explained by the presence of multiple cytological features that can be used to diagnose this type of thyroid carcinoma, we cannot be sure that they are consistently available or sufficiently specific [111]. Pandey et al [103] found that the focal presence of some of these features was the cause of false positive diagnosis for papillary thyroid carcinoma.

4. 6 Bethesda VI category

For category VI "malignant", the malignancy rate varies in the literature between 97% and 100% [106] (table VI).

Table VI: Malignancy rates by Bethesda system category

Bethesda classification	The series				
	Bethesda system [110] (modified by Ali and Cibas)	Bongiovanni et al [112]	Hajmano- -echri et al [89]	Reuters K.B. et al [88]	So Yoan Park et al [106]
I: UNS/ND	1-4 %	16,8%	-	25,7%	9,7%
II: Benin	0-3 %	3,7%	6,9%	6%	2,5%
III: AUS/FLUS	5-15 %	15,9%	50%	12%	37,5%
IV: FN/SFN	15-30 %	26,1%	37%	29,8%	5,7%
V: Suspected of malignancy	60-75 %	75,2%	81,2%	72,5%	100%
VI: Clever	97-99 %	98,6%	100%	97,3%	100%

5 CORRELATION BETWEEN EXTEMPORANEOUS EXAMINATION AND DEFINITIVE HISTOLOGY

Historically, the extemporaneous examination (EE) has been the main means of determining the initial histological diagnosis of a thyroid nodule and therefore guiding the therapeutic strategy. Surgery could be limited to a hemi thyroidectomy in the case of a benign nodule, whereas a malignant diagnosis on EE indicates total thyroidectomy combined with lymph node dissection. Since the advent of CPAF and its establishment as the mainstay of preoperative investigation of thyroid nodules, the role of EE has been widely questioned. The widespread use of the Bethesda system has considerably simplified the diagnostic cytopathology and subsequent management of thyroid nodules. However, cytology alone does not accurately distinguish carcinomas from benign adenomas, particularly in the indeterminate follicular lesions that the Bethesda system has grouped them into categories III and IV. These lesions present a particular risk for over- or under-treatment: an initial lobectomy for a cancer larger than 1 cm may be considered insufficient treatment, while a first total thyroidectomy for a benign nodule may be excessive from an oncological point of view [115].In a retrospective study of 639 patients with indeterminate follicular lesions, Schneider et al [116] found that 9.3% of patients had oncologically inadequate treatment and 19% of patients had oncologically excessive surgery. Category III proved the most problematic for surgeons who struggled to determine the correct extent of initial surgery, with almost 40% of patients receiving inappropriately extensive initial surgery. In this context, EE is still considered by several teams to be a useful tool for optimising decision-making on the initial extent of surgery for indeterminate follicular lesions. In a retrospective study comparing EE and CPAF, Chang et al [117] showed that in the event of disparity between these two diagnostic tools, the accuracy of EE (78.9%) was superior to that of CPAF (21.4%). A positive EE is particularly interesting because of the very low false positive rates of this test, reaching 0% in certain series [118]. Numerous studies have shown that EE has a specificity of over 90% [119, 120]. The high specificity and low false-positive rate of EE mean that total thyroidectomy should be performed in the event of a positive EE result. In a recent large series, Cotton et al [121] showed that, thanks to EE, re-operation was avoided in 8% of patients with lesions in category IV and 2.2% of patients with lesions in category III. Avoiding a second neck operation, with the morbidity that this entails, including the risk of injury to the inferior laryngeal nerve, is the main argument in favour of carrying out EE systematically, and this is particularly true for elderly and frail patients presenting a high anaesthetic risk. However, the true usefulness of EE for indeterminate follicular lesions remains controversial. Indeed, certain histological types, such as vesicular and Hurthle cell carcinomas, NIFT-P and its malignant counterpart FVPTC, may be misdiagnosed by EE [122,123]. Unlike papillary carcinoma, detection of vesicular carcinoma requires complete analysis of the thyroid nodule in order to visualise capsular or vascular invasion to make the diagnosis. In this context, the ability of EE to guide surgery is uncertain given the impossibility of obtaining a correct sample of the capsule to assess invasion [123,124].

A meta-analysis published in 2008, analysing series prior to the Bethesda era, highlighted a high false negative rate for EE and therefore its low sensitivity (67%); the role of EE in guiding the extent of surgery therefore seems limited [125]. Similarly, studies evaluating the role of EE in the post-Bethesda era have confirmed the relatively low sensitivity and NPV of this test. In a retrospective study of 252 patients, Guevara et al [126] reported that EE has a lower sensitivity than CPAF and therefore has a limited impact on surgical strategy. In a recent series, Mallick et al [15] studied 236 patients who had undergone surgery for thyroid nodules with EE; in 95% of cases, EE had no additional benefit and did not change intraoperative management. In 11 patients (4.7%) the initially planned extent of thyroid surgery was modified after the diagnosis made by EE, but this extent was correctly changed in only 5 cases (2.1%). Contrary to the questioning of the usefulness of EE in the case of indeterminate follicular lesions in guiding the intraoperative management of thyroid nodules, this examination is useful in the case of lesions classified in category V by contributing to the determination of the optimal surgical intervention. In a retrospective study conducted at the University of Wisconsin, Haymart et al [127] collected data from patients who had undergone surgery for thyroid nodules over a ten-year period and specifically studied the role of EE for the subgroup of nodules "suspected of malignancy", they found that EE led to the optimal operative procedure in 96% of cases with PPV of 100% and NPV of 85% (Table VII).

Table VII: Sensitivity, specificity, PPV and NPV of EE according to different series

Series	Workforce	Sensitivity	Specific	VPP	VPN
Godey et al [128]	2470	75%	100%	100%	98%
Zhang et al [129]	750	95.50%	100%	100%	
Cerovix et al [130]	675	73%	100%	100%	94%
Mekni et al [131]	1534	67%	99,85%	98%	96,6%
Chao et al [132]	619	82,1%	100%	100%	95,8%

All in all, in this Bethesda era, the contribution of routine EE in cases of indeterminate follicular lesions in guiding surgical strategy appears to be fairly limited. Even if a positive EE is useful and indicates thyroidectomy false negative rates remain high. Furthermore, the potential gain in avoiding two-stage surgery must be balanced against the cost of systematic EE. In this context, there are insufficient arguments to recommend the systematic use of EE for indeterminate follicular lesions, and its use should be limited to cases of cytology classified as Bethesda V, to elderly patients, and to patients at anaesthetic risk for whom any subsequent complementary surgery may pose problems.

CONCLUSION

Thyroid nodules are common pathologies and present a common clinical problem. The challenge in their assessment is to find the right balance between over-treatment and the risk of missing a thyroid cancer. The management of thyroid nodules must be multidisciplinary, involving endocrinologists, radiologists, pathologists and ENT surgeons.Diagnostic strategies were progressively developed in order to minimise the percentage of nodules that had to be managed surgically, so that only suspicious nodules were operated on. Alongside cervical ultrasound, CPAF is the cornerstone of these strategies for exploring thyroid nodules.

REFERENCES

1. Bomeli SR, LeBeau SO, Ferris RL. Evaluation of a thyroid nodule. Otolaryngol Clin North Am. 2010 Apr;43(2):229-38, vii.

2. Popoveniuc G, Jonklaas J. Thyroid nodules. Med Clin North Am. 2012 Mar;96(2):329-49.

3. National Agency for the Development of Medical Evaluation (ANDEM). Diagnostic management of thyroid nodules. Recommendations for clinical practice. Editions Nobert ttali, Paris, 1997.

4. MARTIN HE, ELLIS EB. Biopsy by needle puncture and aspiration. Ann. Surg. 1930; 92: 169-181.

5. Lo Gerfo, P. Coarse-Needle Biopsy of the Thyroid. In: Hamburger, J.I. (eds) Diagnostic Methods in Clinical Thyroidology. Springer, New York, NY.1989

6. Crile, G., Esselstyn, C. B., & Hawk, W. A. (1979). Needle Biopsy in the Diagnosis of Thyroid Nodules Appearing after Radiation. New England Journal of Medicine, 301(18), 997-999.

7. De Micco C. Thyroid cytology: review and prospects. Ann Endocrinol (Paris) 1993; 54: 258-263.

8. Lowhagen T., Grangberg PO., Lundell G. et al. Aspiration biopsy cytology (ABC) in nodules of the thyroid gland suspected to be malignant. Surg Clin North Am 1979; 59: 3-18.

9. Popoveniuc G, Jonklaas J. Thyroid nodules. Med Clin North Am. 2012 Mar; 96(2): 329-49.

10. Pitman M B, Abele J, Ali S Z, Duick D, Elsheikh T M, Jeffrey R B, et al. Technique for thyroid FNA: a synopsis of the National Cancer Institute Thyroid Fine-Needle Aspiration State of the Science Conference. Diagn Cytopathol, 2008, 36(6): p. 407-24.

11. Zajdela A, Zillhardt P, and Voillemot N. Cytological diagnosis by fine needle sampling without aspiration. Cancer, 1987, 59(6): p. 1201-5.

12. Cochand-Priollet B, Vielh P, Royer B, Belleannée G, Collet J F, Goubin-Versini, et al [Thyroid cytopathology: Bethesda System 2010]. Ann Pathol, 2012, 32(3): p. 177-83.

13. Wémeau J-L. Thyroid diseases. 2010. Elsevier Masson.

14. Cibas E S, Alexander E K, Benson C B, de Agustin P P, Doherty G M, Faquin W C, et al. Indications for thyroid FNA and pre-FNA requirements: a synopsis of the National Cancer Institute Thyroid Fine-Needle Aspiration State of the Science Conference. Diagn Cytopathol, 2008,36(6): p. 390-9.

15. Lyle MA, Dean DS: Ultrasound-guided fine-needle aspiration biopsy of

thyroid nodules in patients taking novel oral anticoagulants. Thyroid 2015; 25: 373-6.

16. CARUSO D, MAZZAFERRI E. Fine needle aspiration biopsy in the management of thyroid nodules. Endocrinologist 1991; 1: 194-199].
17. Poulet, G., Massias, J., & Taly, V. (2019). Liquid Biopsy: General Concepts. Acta Cytologica, 1-7.
18. Gharib H, Papini E, Garber J R, Duick D S, Harrel R M, Hegedus L, et al. American association of clinical endocrinologists, American college of endocrinology, and associazione medici endocrinologi medical guidelines for clinical practice for the diagnosis and management of thyroid nodules - 2016 update. Endocrine Practice, 2016, 22(supplement 1): p. 1-60.
19. Haugen B R, Alexander E K, Bible K C, Doherty G M, Mandel S J, Nikiforov Y E, et al. 2015 American Thyroid Association Management Guidelines for Adult Patients with Thyroid Nodules and Differentiated Thyroid Cancer: The American Thyroid Association Guidelines Task Force on Thyroid nodules and Differentiated Thyroid Cancer. Thyroid, 2016, 26(1): p. 1-133.
20. Paschke R, Cantara S, Crescenzi A, Jarzab B, Musholt T J, and Sobrinho Simoes M. European Thyroid Association Guidelines regarding Thyroid Nodule Molecular Fine-Eur Thyroid J, 2017, 6(3): p. 115-129.
21. Russ G, Bonnema S J, Erdogan M F, Durante C, Ngu R, and Leenhardt L. European Thyroid Association Guidelines for Ultrasound Malignancy Risk Stratification of Thyroid Nodules in Adults: The EU-TIRADS. Eur Thyroid J, 2017, 6(5): p. 225-237.
22. Nakamura, H. et al. Is an Increase in Thyroid Nodule Volume a Risk Factor for Malignancy? Thyroid 25, 804-811, doi:10.1089/ thy.2014.0567 (2015).
23. Akhtar, S. & Awan, M. S. Role of fine needle aspiration and frozen section in determining the extent of thyroidectomy. European archives of oto-rhino-laryngology: official journal of the European Federation of Oto-Rhino-Laryngological Societies 264, 1075-1079, doi:10.1007/s00405-007-0302-4 (2007).
24. Erkinuresin, T., & Demirci, H. (2019). Diagnostic accuracy of fine needle aspiration cytology of thyroid nodules. Diagnosis, 0(0).
25. Feldkamp, J., Führer, D., Luster, M., Musholt, T. J., Spitzweg, C., & Schott, M. (2016). Fine Needle Aspiration in the Investigation of Thyroid Nodules. Deutsches Aerzteblatt Online.
26. Schmidkonz, C., Horstrup, K., Weppler, M., Kuwert, T., & Cordes, M. (2018). Fine-needle aspiration biopsies of thyroid nodules. Nuklearmedizin, 57(06), 211-215.

27. Gharib H, Goellner JR, Johnson DA. Fine-needle aspiration cytology of the thyroid: a 12-year experience with 11,000 biopsies. Clin Lab Med. 1993;13:699-709.

28. LAYFIELD L, LONES M. Necrosis in thyroid nodules after fine needle aspiration biobsy. Report of two cases. Acta cytol 1991; 35: 427-430.

29. Ito Y, Tomoda C, Uruno T, et al: Needle tract implantation of papillary thyroid carcinoma after fine-needle aspiration biopsy. World J Surg 2005; 29: 1544-9.

30. Cannoni M, Demard F, Bourdinière A, et al. Extemporaneous biopsy and its consequences. In: Les nodules thyroïdiens, du diagnostic à la chirurgie. Rapport Soc. Française d'ORL et de pathologie cervico-faciale. Arnette Edition (Paris); 1995, 205-11.

31. Garrel R, Périé S. Epidemiology of thyroid pathologies. In: Pathologies chirurgicales de la glande thyroïde. Rapport Soc. Française d'ORL et de chirurgie de la face et du cou. SFORL Edition (Paris); 2012, 61-74.

32. Chan JKC. Tumors of the thyroid and parathyroid glands. In: Fletcher 3rd CHDM, editor. Diagnostic histopathology oftumors. 2 Churchill: Livingstone Elsevier; 2007. p. 997-1079.

33. Alexander EK. Approach to the patient with a cytologically indeterminate thyroid nodule. J Clin Endocrinol Metab 2008; 93: 4175-82.

34. Bair ND, Hahn PF, Gervais DA, et al. Fine-needle aspiration biopsy of thyroid nodules: experience in a cohort of 944 patients. AJR Am J Roentgenol 2009; 193: 1175-9.

35. Seningen JL, Nassar A, Henry MR. Correlation of thyroid nodule fine-needle aspiration cytology with corresponding histology at Mayo Clinic, 2001-2007: an institutional experience of 1945 cases. Diagn Cytopathol 2012; 40(suppl. 1): E27-32.

36. Ali SZ, Cibas ES 2009 The Bethesda System for Reporting Thyroid Cytopathology: Definitions, Criteria and Explanatory Notes. Springer, New York, NY.

37. Cibas ES, Ali SZ 2009 The Bethesda System for Reporting Thyroid Cytopathology. Thyroid 19:1159-1165.

38. Haugen BR, Alexander EK, Bible KC, Doherty GM, Mandel J, Nikiforov YE, Pacini F, Randolph GW, Sawka AM, Schlumberger M, Schuff KG, Sherman SI, Sosa JA, Steward DL, Tuttle RM, Wartofsky L 2016 2015 American Thyroid Association management guidelines for adult patients with thyroid nodules and differentiated thyroid cancer: the American Thyroid Association Guidelines Task Force on Thyroid Nodules and Differentiated

Thyroid Cancer. Thyroid 26:1-133.
39. Renshaw AA 2012 Histologic follow-up of nondiagnostic thyroid fine needle aspirations: implications for adequacy criteria. Diagn Cytopathol 40: E13-15.

40. Vivero M, Renshaw AA, Krane JF 2017 Adequacy criteria for thyroid FNA evaluated by ThinPrep slides only. Cancer 125:534-543.
41. Cochand-Priollet B and Vielh P. Special issue "Cytopathology". Ann Pathol, 2012, 36(6): p. el-2, 387-8.
42. Cochand-Priollet B, Vielh P, Royer B, Belleannée G, Collet J-F, Goubin-Versini I, et al. Thyroid cytopathology: the 2010 Bethesda system. Annales de Pathologie, 2012, 32(3): p. 177-183.
43. Renshaw AA 2002 "Histiocytoid" cells in fine-needle aspirations of papillary carcinoma of the thyroid: frequency and significance of an under- recognized cytologic pattern. Cancer 96:240-243.
44. Yang GC, Stern CM, Messina AV 2010 Cystic papillary thyroid carcinoma in fine needle aspiration may represent a subset of the encapsulated variant in WHO classification. Diagn Cytopathol 38:721-726.
45. Kelman AS, Rathan A, Leibowitz J, Burstein DE, Haber RS 2001 Thyroid cytology and the risk of malignancy in thyroid nodules: importance of nuclear atypia in indeterminate specimens. Thyroid 11:271-277.
46. Yang J, Schnadig V, Logrono R, Wasserman PG 2007 Fine-needle aspiration of thyroid nodules: a study of 4703 patients with histologic and clinical correlations. Cancer 111:306-315.
47. Ali S, Cibas E 2018 The Bethesda System for Reporting Thyroid Cytopathology: Definitions, Criteria, and Explanatory Notes. Second edition. Springer, New York, NY.
48. Faquin WC, Wong LQ, Afrogheh AH, Ali SZ, Bishop JA, Bongiovanni M, Pusztaszeri MP, VandenBussche CJ, Gourmaud J, Vaickus LJ, Baloch ZW 2016 Impact of reclassifying noninvasive follicular variant of papillary thyroid carcinoma on the risk of malignancy in The Bethesda System for Reporting Thyroid Cytopathology. Cancer Cytopathol 124:181-187.
49. Strickland KC, Howitt BE, Marqusee E, Alexander EK, Cibas ES, Krane JF, Barletta JA 2015 The impact of noninvasive follicular variant of papillary thyroid carcinoma on rates of malignancy for fine-needle aspiration diagnostic categories. Thyroid 25:987-992.
50. Krane JF, Alexander EK, Cibas ES, Barletta JA 2016 Coming to terms with NIFTP: a provisional approach for cytologists. Cancer Cytopathol 124:767- 772.
51. Pusztaszeri M, Rossi ED, Auger M, Baloch Z, Bishop J, Bongiovanni M,

Chandra A, Cochand-Priollet B, Fadda G, Hirokawa M, Hong S, Kakudo K, Krane JF, Nayar R, Parangi S, Schmitt F, Faquin WC 2016 The Bethesda System for Reporting Thyroid Cytopathology: proposed modifications and updates for the second edition from an international panel. Acta Cytol 60:399-405.

52. Sohn YM, Kim MJ, Kim EK, Kwak JY. Diagnostic performance of thyroglobulin value in indeterminate range in fine needle aspiration washout fluid from lymph nodes of thyroid cancer. Yonsei medical journal. 2012; 53(1):126-31. doi: 10.3349/ymj.2012.53.1.126 PMID: 22187242; PubMed Central PMCID: PMC3250316.
53. Thomas, C. M., Asa, S. L., Ezzat, S., Sawka, A. M., & Goldstein, D. (2019). Diagnosis and pathologic characteristics of medullary thyroid carcinoma-review of current guidelines. Current Oncology, 26(5).
54. De Micco C., Zoro P., Henry JF. Markers of malignancy in cytopunction of thyroid nodules. Ann Pathol 1994; 14: 378-383.
55. Flament JB, Delisle MJ, Pluot M. Management of the isolated thyroid nodule: cytological evaluation. Accords et controverses. Ann Endocrinol (Paris) 1993; 54: 264-268.
56. Franc B, Allery Y., Hejblum G. Cytopuncture of thyroid tumours. Rev Prat 1996; 46: 2315-2320.
57. Najafian, A., Noureldine, S., Azar, F., Atallah, C., Trinh, G., Schneider, E. B. Zeiger, M. A. (2017). RASMutations, andRET/PTCandPAX8/PPAR-gammaChromosomal Rearrangements Are Also Prevalent in Benign Thyroid Lesions: Implications Thereof and A Systematic Review. Thyroid, 27(1), 39-48.
58. Fonesca E., Eloy C., Sobrinho-Simoes M. Well-differentiated vesicular tumours: new molecular concepts? New diagnostic criteria? Bulletin de la Division Française de l'AIP 2007; 45: 20-24.
59. Sobrinho-Simoes M., Preto A., Rocha AS. Molecular pathology of well differentiated thyroid carcinoma. Virchows Arch 2005; 447: 787_93.
60. Khan, M. S., Qadri, Q., Makhdoomi, M. J., Wani, M. A., Malik, A. A., Niyaz, M.,Mudassar, S. (2018). RET/PTC Gene Rearrangements in Thyroid Carcinogenesis: Assessment and Clinico-Pathological Correlations. Pathology & Oncology Research.
61. Rocha AS., Soares P., Seruca R. et al. Abnormalities of the E-cadherin / catenin adhesion complex in classical papillary thyroid carcinoma and its diffuse sclerosing variant. J Pathol 2001; 194: 358-366.
62. Zhu X, Wang X, Gong Y, Deng J. E-cadherin on epithelial-mesenchymal transition in thyroid cancer. Cancer Cell Int. 2021 Dec 20;21(1):695.

63. Zhu Z., Ghandi M., Nikiforova MN., Fisher AH., Nikiforov YE. Molecular profile and clinical pathologic features of the follicular variant of papillary thyroid carcinoma. An usually high prevalence of ras mutations. Am J Clin Pathol 2003; 120: 71-77.
64. Lectère J., Orgiazzi J., Rousset B., Schlienger JL., Wemeau JL. In: La thyroïde, Ed. Elsevier 2001, 2nd Edition.

65. Cochand-Priollet B., Pratt JJ., Polivka M. et al. Thyroid fine-needle aspiration: the morphological features on thin prep slide preparations. Eighty cases with histological control. Cytopathology 2003; 14: 343-349.
66. Mahajan S, Rajwanshi A, Srinivasan R, Radotra BD, Panda N. Should Liquid Based Cytology (LBC) be Applied to Thyroid Fine Needle Aspiration Cytology Samples? Comparative Analysis of Conventional and LBC Smears. J Cytol. 2021 Oct-Dec;38(4):198-202.
67. Ben Abdelkrim S, Rammel S, Ben yacoub Abid L, Abdelkefi M, Ben Ali M, and Mokni M. L'examen extemporané en pathologie thyroïdienne: interet et limites. Journal Africain du Cancer / African Journal of cancer, 2012, 4 (3): p. 171-175.
68. StanCiu-PoP C, PoP F C, thiry a, SCagnol i, Maweja S, haMmoir e, et al. Interests and limitations of extemporaneous examination in thyroid pathology systematic review of the literature and evidence-based assessment. Rev Med Liège 2015, 70 (12): p. 683-643.
69. Wei S. Oncocytic (Hürthle cell) tumors. PathologyOutlines.com website. https://www.pathologyoutlines.com/topic/thyroidhurthle.html.
70. Esserman LJ, Thompson IM, Reid B, et al. Addressing overdiagnosis and overtreatment in cancer: a prescription for change. Lancet Oncol 2014;15: e234-42.
71. Baloch ZW, Shafique K, Flanagan M, et al. Encapsulated classic and follicular variants of papillary thyroid carcinoma: comparative clinicopathologic study. Endocr Pract 2010;16:952-9.
72. Nikiforov YE, Seethala RR, Tallini G, et al. Nomenclature Revision for Encapsulated Follicular Variant of Papillary Thyroid Carcinoma: A Paradigm Shift to Reduce Overtreatment of Indolent Tumors. JAMA Oncol 2016;2:1023-9.
73. Nikiforov YE, Baloch ZW, Hodak SP, et al. Change in Diagnostic Criteria for Noninvasive Follicular Thyroid Neoplasm With Papillarylike Nuclear Features. JAMA Oncol 2018;4:1125-6.
74. Cho U, Mete O, Kim MH, et al. Molecular correlates and rate of lymph node metastasis of non-invasive follicular thyroid neoplasm with papillary-like

nuclear features and invasive follicular variant papillary thyroid carcinoma: the impact of rigid criteria to distinguish non-invasive follicular thyroid neoplasm with papillary-like nuclear features. Mod Pathol 2017; 30:810-25.
75. Kim TH, Lee M, Kwon AY, et al. Molecular genotyping of the non-invasive encapsulated follicular variant of papillary thyroid carcinoma. Histopathology 2018;72:648-61.

76. Xu B, Tallini G, Scognamiglio T, et al. Outcome of Large Noninvasive Follicular Thyroid Neoplasm with PapillaryLike Nuclear Features. Thyroid 2017;27:512-7.
77. Haugen BR, Sawka AM, Alexander EK, et al. American Thyroid Association Guidelines on the Management of Thyroid Nodules and Differentiated Thyroid Cancer Task Force Review and Recommendation on the Proposed Renaming of Encapsulated Follicular Variant Papillary Thyroid Carcinoma Without Invasion to Noninvasive Follicular Thyroid Neoplasm with Papillary-Like Nuclear Features. Thyroid 2017;27:481-3.
78. Andrey Bychkov. Papillary carcinoma [cited 2018-02-15]; Available from: http://www.pathologyoutlines.com/imgau/thyroidbychkov11.JPG.
79. Kondo T, Nakazawa T, Murata S, and Katoh R. Stromal elastosis in papillary thyroid carcinomas. Hum Pathol, 2005, 36(5): p. 474_9.
80. Badawy M and Wafaey F. Follicular carcinoma [cited 2018-02-02]; available from:
http://www.pathologyoutlines.com/imgau/thyroidfollicularPathout01.jpg
81. Andrey Bychkov. Follicular carcinoma. 2017 [cited 2018-02-15]; Available from: http://www.pathologyoutlines.com/imgau/thyroidbychkov5.JPG
82. Erickson L A. Atlas of Endocrine Pathology 2014. Springer Science & Business Media.
83. Lew J I, Snyder R A, Sanchez Y M, and Solorzano C C. Fine needle aspiration of the thyroid: correlation with final histopathology in a surgical series of 797 patients. J Am Coll Surg, 2011,213(1): p. 188-94; discussion 194-5.
84. Gharib H, Papini E, Garber JR, Duick DS, Harrell RM, Hegedus L, Paschke R, Valcavi R, Vitti P 2016 AMERICAN ASSOCIATION OF CLINICAL ENDOCRINOLOGISTS, AMERICAN COLLEGE OF ENDOCRINOLOGY, AND ASSOCIAZIONE MEDICI ENDOCRINOLOGI MEDICAL GUIDELINES FOR CLINICAL PRACTICE FOR THE DIAGNOSIS AND MANAGEMENT OF THYROID NODULES--2016 UPDATE. Endocrine practice: official journal of the American College of Endocrinology and the American Association of Clinical Endocrinologists. 2016; 22:622-639.

85. Haugen BR, Alexander EK, Bible KC, Doherty GM, Mandel SJ, Nikiforov YE, Pacini F, Randolph GW, Sawka AM, Schlumberger M, Schuff KG, Sherman SI, Sosa JA, Steward DL, Tuttle RM, Wartofsky L 2016 2015 American Thyroid Association Management Guidelines for Adult Patients with Thyroid Nodules and Differentiated Thyroid Cancer: The American Thyroid Association Guidelines Task Force on Thyroid Nodules and Differentiated Thyroid Cancer. Thyroid: official journal of the American Thyroid Association 26:1-133.
86. Bongiovanni, M., Spitale, A., Faquin, W. C., Mazzucchelli, L., & Baloch, Z. W. (2012). The Bethesda System for Reporting Thyroid Cytopathology: A Meta-Analysis. Acta Cytologica, 56(4), 333-339.
87. Bongiovanni M, Spitale A, Faquin W C, Mazzucchelli L, and Baloch Z W. The Bethesda System for Reporting Thyroid Cytopathology: a meta- analysis. Acta Cytol, 2012,56(4): p. 333-9.
88. Reuters, K. B., Mamone, M. C. O. C., Ikejiri, E. S., Camacho, C. P., Nakabashi, C. C. D., Janovsky, C. C. P. S., ... Biscolla, R. P. M. (2018). Bethesda Classification and Cytohistological Correlation of Thyroid Nodules in a Brazilian Thyroid Disease Center. European Thyroid Journal, 7(3), 133-138.
89. Hajmanoochehri F and Rabiee E. FNAC accuracy in diagnosis of thyroid neoplasms considering all diagnostic categories of the Bethesda reporting system: A single-institute experience. Journal of Cytology / Indian Academy of Cytologists, 2015,32(4): p. 238-243.
90. Muratli A, Erdogan N, Sevim S, Unal I, Akyuz S. Diagnostic efficacy and importance of fine-needle aspiration cytology of thyroid nodules. J Cytol. 2014;31:73-8.
91. Anand, B., Ramdas, A., Ambroise, M. M., & Kumar, N. P. (2020). The Bethesda System for Reporting Thyroid Cytopathology: A Cytohistological Study. Journal of Thyroid Research, 2020, 1-8.
92. Seiberling KA D J a G J. Ultrasound-guided fine needle aspiration biopsy of thyroid nodules performed in the offce. Laryngoscope, 2008,118(2): p. 228-231. 5 Ohori NP, Nikiforova MN, Schoedel KE, LeBeau SO, Hodak SP, Seethala RR, Carty SE, Ogilvie JB, Yip L, Nikiforov YE. Contribution of molecular testing to thyroid fine-needle aspiration cytology of "follicular lesion of undetermined significance/atypia of undetermined significance". Cancer Cytopathol. 2010; 118(1):17-23.
93. Esmaili H A and Taghipour H. Fine-Needle Aspiration in the Diagnosis of Thyroid Diseases: An Appraisal in Our Institution. ISRN Pathology, 2012, p. 4.
94. Wong LQ, Baloch ZW. Analysis of the Bethesda system for reporting

thyroid cytopathology and similar precursor thyroid cytopathology reporting schemes. Adv Anat Pathol. 2012;19:313-9.
95. Yang J, Schnadig V, Logrono R, and Wasserman P G. Fine-needle aspiration of thyroid nodules: a study of 4703 patients with histologic and clinical correlations. Cancer, 2007,111(5): p. 306-15.

96. Ali SZ: Thyroid cytopathology: Bethesda and beyond. Acta Cytol 2011; 55: 4-12.
97. Kim SK, Hwang TS, Yoo YB, Han HS, Kim DL, Song KH, Lim SD, Kim WS, Paik NS: Surgical results of thyroid nodules according to a management guideline based on the braf(v600e) mutation status. J Clin Endocrinol Metabol 2011; 96: 658-664.
98. Guo, Y. Kaminoh, T. Forward, F. L. Schwartz, and S. Jenkinson, "Fine needle aspiration of thyroid nodules using the bethesda system for reporting thyroid cytopathology: an institutional experience in a rural setting," International Journal of Endocrinology, vol. 2017, Article ID 9601735, 6 pages, 2017.
99. S. Mondal, S. Sinha, B. Basak, D. Roy, and S. Sinha, "(e Bethesda system for reporting thyroid fine needle aspirates: a cytologic study with histologic follow-up," Journal of Cytology, vol. 30, no. 2, pp. 94-99, 2013.
100. Ali SZ, Cibas ES: The Bethesda System for Reporting Thyroid Cytopathology. Definitions, criteria and explanatory notes. New York, Springer, 2010.
101. Cooper DS, Doherty GM, Haugen BR, Kloos RT, Lee SL, Mandel SJ, Mazzaferri EL, McIver B, Pacini F, Schlumberger M, Sherman SI, Steward DL, Tuttle RM: Revised American Thyroid Association management guidelines for patients with thyroid nodules and differentiated thyroid cancer. Thyroid 2009; 19: 1167-1214.
102. Agcaoglu O, Aksakal N, Ozcinar B, Sarici IS, Ercan G, Kucukyilmaz M, et al. Factors that affect the false-negative outcomes of fine-needle aspiration biopsy in thyroid nodules. Int J Endocrinol 2013. 2013 126084.
103. Pandey P, Dixit A, Mahajan NC. Fine-needle aspiration of the thyroid: A cytohistologic correlation with critical evaluation of discordant cases. Thyroid Res Pract. 2012;9:32-9.
104. Sinna EA, Ezzat N. Diagnostic accuracy of fine needle aspiration cytology in thyroid lesions. J Egypt Natl Canc Inst. 2012;24:63-70.
105. Cibas E S and Ali S Z. The Bethesda System For Reporting Thyroid Cytopathology. Am J Clin Pathol, 2009,132(5): p. 658-65.
106. Park S Y, Hahn S Y, Shin J H, Ko E Y, and Oh Y L. The Diagnostic

Performance of Thyroid US in Each Category of the Bethesda System for Reporting Thyroid Cytopathology. PLoS ONE, 2016,11(6).
107. Cibas ES, Ali SZ. NCI Thyroid FNA State of the Science Conference. The Bethesda system for reporting thyroid cytopathology. Am J Clin Pathol. 2009;132:658-65.

108. Schreiner AM, Yang GC. Adenomatoid nodules are the main cause for discrepant histology in 234 thyroid fine-needle aspirates reported as follicular neoplasm. Diagn Cytopathol. 2012;40:375-9.
109. Yang J, Schnadig V, Logrono R, Wasserman PG. Fine-needle aspiration of thyroid nodules: A study of 4703 patients with histologic and clinical correlations. Cancer. 2007;111:306-15.
110. Ali SZ, Cibas ES: The Bethesda System for Reporting Thyroid Cytopathology. Definitions, criteria and explanatory notes. New York, Springer, 2010.
111. Chandanwale SS, Kumar H, Buch AC, Vimal SS, Soraisham P. Papillary thyroid carcinoma, a diagnostic approach in fine needle aspiration: Review of literature. Clin Cancer Investig J. 2013;2:339-43.
112. Bongiovanni, M., Spitale, A., Faquin, W. C., Mazzucchelli, L., & Baloch, Z.
W. (2012). The Bethesda System for Reporting Thyroid Cytopathology: A Meta-Analysis. Acta Cytologica, 56(4), 333-339.
113. Gharib H, Papini E, Garber JR, Duick DS, Harrell RM, Hegedüs L, Paschke R, Valcavi R, Vitti P. AACE/ACE/AME task force on thyroid nodules, American association of clinical endocrinologists, American college of endocrinology, and Associazione Medici Endocrinologi medical guidelines for clinical practice for the diagnosis and management of thyroid Nodules- 2016 update. Endocr Pract. 2016;22(5):622-39.
114. Ho AS, Sarti EE, Jain KS, Wang H, Nixon IJ, Shaha AR, Shah JP, Kraus DH, Ghossein R, Fish SA, Wong RJ, Lin O, Morris LG. Malignancy rate in thyroid nodules classified as Bethesda category III (AUS/FLUS). Thyroid. 2014;24(5): 832-9.
115. Haugen BR, Alexander EK, Bible KC, et al. 2015 American Thyroid Association Management Guidelines for Adult Patients with Thyroid Nodules and Differentiated Thyroid Cancer: The American Thyroid Association Guidelines Task Force on Thyroid Nodules and Differentiated Thyroid Cancer. Thyroid 2016; 26:1-133.
116. Schneider DF, Cherney Stafford LM, Brys N, et al. Gauging the extent of thyroidectomy for indeterminate thyroid nodules: an oncologic perspective.

Endocr Pract 2017; 23:442-50.
117. Chang HY, Lin JD, Chen JF, et al. Correlation of fine needle aspiration cytology and frozen section biopsies in the diagnosis of thyroid nodules. J Clin Pathol 1997;50:1005-9.
118. Kennedy JM, Robinson RA. Thyroid Frozen Sections in Patients With Preoperative FNAs: Review of Surgeons' Preoperative Rationale, Intraoperative Decisions, and Final Outcome. Am J Clin Pathol 2016; 145:660-5.

119. Cohen MA, Patel KR, Gromis J, et al. Retrospective evaluation of frozen section use for thyroid nodules with a prior fine needle aspiration diagnosis of Bethesda II-VI: The Weill Cornell Medical College experience. World J Otorhinolaryngol Head Neck Surg 2015; 1:5-10.
120. Huber GF, Dziegielewski P, Matthews TW, et al. Intraoperative frozen-section analysis for thyroid nodules: a step toward clarity or confusion? Arch Otolaryngol Head Neck Surg 2007; 133:874-81.
121. Cotton TM, Xin J, Sandyhya J, et al. Frozen section analysis in the post-Bethesda era. J Surg Res 2016; 205:393-7.
122. Antic T, Taxy JB. Thyroid frozen section: supplementary or unnecessary? Am J Surg Pathol 2013;37:282-6.
123. Udelsman R, Westra WH, Donovan PI, et al. Randomized prospective evaluation of frozen-section analysis for follicular neoplasms of the thyroid. Ann Surg 2001; 233:716-22.
124. Carling T, Udelsman R. Follicular neoplasms of the thyroid: what to recommend. Thyroid 2005;15:583-7.
125. Peng Y, Wang HH. A meta-analysis of comparing fineneedle aspiration and frozen section for evaluating thyroid nodules. Diagn Cytopathol 2008; 36:916-20.
126. Guevara N, Lassalle S, Benaim G, et al. Role of frozen section analysis in nodular thyroid pathology. Eur Ann Otorhinolaryngol Head Neck Dis 2015; 132:67-70.
127. Haymart MR, Greenblatt DY, Elson DF, et al. The role of intraoperative frozen section if suspicious for papillary thyroid cancer. Thyroid 2008; 18:419-23.
128. Godey B, Le Clech G, Inigues JP, Legall F, Beust L, Bourdiniére J. L'examen anatomo-pathologique extemporané dans la chirurgie des cancers thyroïdiens: intérêts et limites. Ann Otolaryngol Chir Cervicofac 1996; 113: 219-24.
129. Zhang L, Li W, Jin M.- The value of frozen section examination in thyroid surgery. Lin Chung Er Bi Yan Hou Tou Jing Wai Ke Za Zhi, 2007, 21, 299-

301.
130. Cerovix S, Ignjatovic M, Brajuskovic G, et al - The value of intraoperative diagnosis in thyroid surgery. Arch Oncol, 2004, 12, 48.
131. Mekni A, Limaiem F, Cherif K, et al - Value of intraoperative frozen-section analysis in thyroid surgery. Presse Med, 2008, 37, 949-955.
132. Chao TC, Lin JD, Chao HH, et al - Surgical treatment of solitary thyroid nodules via fine-needle aspiration biopsy and frozen-section analysis. Ann Surg Oncol, 2007, 14, 712-718.

APPENDICES

Appendix I:EU-TIRADS classification (2017) [21]

Category	US features	Malignancy risk, %
EU-TIRADS 1: normal	No nodules	None
EU-TIRADS 2: benign	Pure cyst Entirely spongiform	≅0
EU-TIRADS 3: low risk	Ovoid, smooth isoechoic/hyperechoic No features of high suspicion	2–4
EU-TIRADS 4: intermediate risk	Ovoid, smooth, mildly hypoechoic No features of high suspicion	6–17
EU-TIRADS 5: high risk	At least 1 of the following features of high suspicion: - Irregular shape - Irregular margins - Microcalcifications - Marked hypoechogenicity (and solid)	26–87

EU-TIRADS, European Thyroid Imaging Reporting and Data System; US, ultrasound.

Appendix II: Bethesda classification (2017) [47]

Catégorie	Description et traitement	Risque de malignité
Bethesda I <10% des cas	• Biopsie non diagnostic ou non satisfaisant: échantillon inadéquat avec un nombre insuffisant de cellules folliculaires. • Répéter la ponction à l'aiguille fine (PAF) écho-guidée	-
Bethesda II 65%	• Bénin, compatible avec un adenome folliculaire: Tissu thyroïdien normal présentant des nodules de goitres adénomateux ou multinodulaires • Pas d'investigation ultérieure neccessaire si le nodule reste stable. Par contre une croissance de plus de 50% du volume des nodules ou de 20% dans au moins deux dimensions des nodules est considérée comme cliniquement significative et dans ce cas il faut refaire la ponction à l'aiguille fine ou des échographies en séries. En cas de suspicion de malignité il faut procéder à une chirurgie diagnostique.[5][6][7]	0-3%
Bethesda III 10%	• Atypie ou lésions folliculaire de signification indéterminée: les lésions ne sont pas bénignes de manière convaincante • Refaire la PAF dans trois à six mois ou operer selon la situation clinique	5-15%
Bethesda IV	• Néoplasie folliculaire ou suspect de néoplasie folliculaire: comprend les adénomes microfolliculaires ou cellulaires • Indication opératoire, généralement sans examen extemporané. la distinction entre adénome et carcinome est impossible à la cytologie. Pour le diagnostic final, il faut analyser en totalité la capsule du nodule à la recherche d'invasions transcapsulaire ou d'invasion vasculaire	15-30%
Bethesda V	• suspect de malignité: les lésions avec des caractéristiques de malignité qui ne sont pas définies pour le cancer de la thyroïde • Opération avec examens extemporanés	60-75%
Bethesda VI	• Malin: lésions caractéristiques du cancer de la thyroïde exemple pour les cancers papillaires, on a de grandes cellules avec un cytoplasme en verre dépoli, des nucléoles proéminents et des inclusions cytoplasmiques intranucléaires. Tandis que le cancer médullaire montre des cellules dispersées avec des noyaux excentriquement déplacés et un cytoplasme légèrement granulaire généralement configuré comme une larme. • Opération sans examens extemporané	97-99%

Annex III: WHO classification of malignant thyroid tumours 2017 [31]

WHO classification of tumours of the thyroid gland (2017)

Follicular adenoma
Hyalinizing trabecular tumour
Other encapsulated follicular-patterned thyroid tumours
- Follicular tumour of uncertain malignant potential
- Well-differentiated tumour of uncertain malignant potential
- Noninvasive follicular thyroid neoplasm with papillary-like nuclear features

Papillary thyroid carcinoma (PTC)
- Papillary carcinoma
- Follicular variant of PTC
- Encapsulated variant of PTC
- Papillary microcarcinoma
- Columnar cell variant of PTC
- Oncocytic variant of PTC

Follicular thyroid carcinoma (FTC), NOS
- FTC, minimally invasive
- FTC, encapsulated angioinvasive
- FTC, widely invasive

Hürthle (oncocytic) cell tumours
- Hürthle cell adenoma
- Hürthle cell carcinoma

Poorly differentiated thyroid carcinoma
Anaplastic thyroid carcinoma
Squamous cell carcinoma
Medullary thyroid carcinoma
Mixed medullary and follicular thyroid carcinoma
Mucoepidermoid carcinoma
Sclerosing mucoepidermoid carcinoma with eosinophilia
Mucinous carcinoma
Ectopic thymoma
Spindle epithelial tumour with thymus-like differentiation
Intrathyroid thymic carcinoma

Paraganglioma and mesenchymal/stromal tumours
- Paraganglioma
- Peripheral nerve sheath tumours (PNSTs)
  - Schwannoma
  - Malignant PNST
- Benign vascular tumours
  - Haemangioma
  - Cavernous haemangioma
  - Lymphangioma
- Angiosarcoma
- Smooth muscle tumours
  - Leiomyoma
  - Leiomyosarcoma
- Solitary fibrous tumour

Hematolymphoid tumours
- Langerhans cell histiocytosis
- Rosai-Dorfman disease
- Follicular dendritic cell sarcoma
- Primary thyroid lymphoma

Germ cell tumours
- Benign teratoma
- Immature teratoma
- Malignant teratoma

Secondary tumours

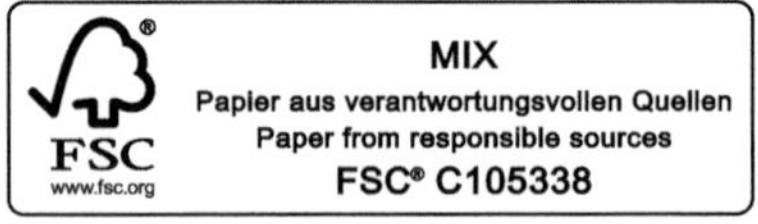

Printed by Books on Demand GmbH, Norderstedt / Germany